I0005519

# 40 Meal Recipes to Consider after You Quit Smoking:

## Control the Cravings with Proper Nutrition and a Healthy Diet

## By

## Joe Correa CSN

# COPYRIGHT

This publication is designed to provide accurate and authoritative information in regard to the subject matter covered. It is sold with the understanding that neither the author nor the publisher is engaged in rendering medical advice. If medical advice or assistance is needed, consult with a doctor. This book is considered a guide and should not be used in any way detrimental to your health. Consult with a physician before starting this nutritional plan to make sure it's right for you.

## ACKNOWLEDGEMENTS

This book is dedicated to my friends and family that have had mild or serious illnesses so that you may find a solution and make the necessary changes in your life.

# 40 Meal Recipes to Consider after You Quit Smoking:

## Control the Cravings with Proper Nutrition and a Healthy Diet

## By

## Joe Correa CSN

# CONTENTS

## ABOUT THE AUTHOR

After years of Research, I honestly believe in the positive effects that proper nutrition can have over the body and mind. My knowledge and experience has helped me live healthier throughout the years and which I have shared with family and friends. The more you know about eating and drinking healthier, the sooner you will want to change your life and eating habits.

Nutrition is a key part in the process of being healthy and living longer so get started today. The first step is the most important and the most significant.

# INTRODUCTION

40 Meal Recipes to Consider after You Quit Smoking: Control the Cravings with Proper Nutrition and a Healthy Diet

By Joe Correa CSN

There are a lot of published studies on how smoking affects our physical and mental health. Anxiety, headaches, hunger, and concentration disorder are just some of the symptoms.

Making the decision to quit smoking is probably the best one you have ever made, in your entire life. Being aware of the damage smoking can cause unfortunately is not enough to force us to make this vital decision. The key lies in our head and how strongly are we dedicated to throwing away what's harming us and to live a long and healthy life.

However, an important issue related to this problem is a myth we've often heard: "If I quit smoking, I will probably start gaining weight! The problem is that all smokers are used to having something in their hands and mouth, and when they quit smoking, they turn to unhealthy snacks to keep their hands and mouth busy. This habit, naturally, leads to gaining weight, which is again related to smoking.

Food cravings are at its peak in the first few weeks of recovery. This is a crucial time to trick your organism and eliminate those feelings.

Food cravings are not a mistery. Physicians and nutritionists agree that <u>the type of food you eat determines the amount of food cravings you have</u>. Whole, healthy foods with plenty of fruits, vegetables, nuts, and seeds, are proven to reduce food cravings. Healthy carbs full of fiber and natural sugar will keep your glucose levels in check and your appetite under control.

This book offers you exactly that! Plenty of healthy recipes that will definitely control your food cravings and keep your organism balanced. The recipes inside like: "Barley Porridge" or "Green Apple Overnight Oats with Raisins" are full of precious fibers and the perfect way to start your new, healthy, and smoke-free day.

I have combined some amazingly nutritious ingredients but I also combined them in a delicious way. Once you have tried: "Stewed Beef with Olives" or "Southern Lamb Stew", you will be preparing these recipes for years to come. They are simple, extremely healthy, and surpisingly easy to make.

By starting to prepare these recipes you are almost at the point where health problems, bad breath, and breathing problems are things of the past. You quit smoking! And I would really like to take this opportunity to say "congratulations!" You're one of the few people who has a strong will! You should be proud of yourself! My book is here to help you improve your overall health and give your body the easiest way to overcome cravings.

# 40 MEAL RECIPES TO CONSIDER AFTER YOU QUIT SMOKING: CONTROL THE CRAVINGS WITH PROPER NUTRITION AND A HEALTHY DIET

## 1. Creamy Avocado and Flaxseed Oats

**Ingredients:**

½ avocado, peeled

1 large kiwi, peeled and sliced

2 cups of skim milk

½ cup of rolled oats

1 tbsp of flaxseed

**Preparation:**

Place oats in a serving bowl. Add one cup of milk and set aside to soak for ten minutes.

Meanwhile, place kiwi, avocado, and the remaining cup of milk in a food processor. Pulse briefly to combine.

Transfer to a serving bowl and stir well to combine with oats. Sprinkle with flaxseed and serve.

This recipe is also a great option for overnight oats. Prepare the night before and refrigerate overnight. Serve cold.

Nutrition information per serving: Kcal: 420, Protein: 13.5g, Carbs: 64.2g, Fats: 21.5g

## 2. Barley Porridge

**Ingredients:**

½ cup of barley, cooked

1 cup of almond milk

1 tbsp of honey

a handful of fresh dates, finely chopped

1 tbsp of fresh lemon juice

1 tbsp of almonds, finely chopped

**Preparation:**

Soak barley overnight. Drain and place in a deep pot. Add about two cups of water and bring it to a boil. Cook for 15 minutes over medium temperature. Remove from the heat, drain and cool for a while.

Transfer to a powerful food procesoor. Add fresh dates and pulse until well incorporated.

Place in a serving bowl, add almond milk, one tablespoon of lemon juice, and top with finely chopped almonds. Stir in one tablespoon of honey and serve.

Nutrition information per serving: Kcal: 172, Protein: 15.5g, Carbs: 48.8g, Fats: 1.2g

## 3. Greek Yogurt with Cranberries

**Ingredients:**

1 ½ cup of Greek yogurt

1 large banana

¼ cup of cranberries

1 tsp of vanilla sugar

1 tbsp of honey

**Preparation:**

Peel and roughly chop the banana. Mash well with a fork and transfer to a food processor. Add Greek yogurt, vanilla sugar, and honey. Pulse well to combine and pour into a bowl.

Stir in cranberries and serve.

Nutrition information per serving: Kcal: 199, Protein: 17g, Carbs: 31.2g, Fats: 8.6g

## 4. Green Apple Overnight Oats with Raisins

**Ingredients:**

4 tbsp of rolled oats

1 tbsp of raisins

1 cup of skim milk

1 small green apple, peeled and chopped

1 tbsp of honey

**Preparation:**

In a medium-sized bowl, combine rolled oats with milk. Stir in honey and refrigerate overnight.

Stir in one tablespoon of raisins and top with chopped apple before serving.

You can add about ½ tsp of cinnamon, but this is optional.

Nutrition information per serving: Kcal: 322, Protein: 7.3g, Carbs: 60.6g, Fats: 8.1g

## 5. Matcha Banana Pudding

**Ingredients:**

2 large bananas, peeled and chopped

1 ½ tsp of Matcha

1 cup of Greek yogurt (can be replaced with almond yogurt)

2 tbsp of honey

2 tbsp of freshly squeezed lemon juice

**Preparation:**

Combine the ingredients in a food processor and mix for 30 seconds.

Place the mixture in a bowl and refrigerate overnight.

Serve cold.

Nutrition information per serving: Kcal: 195, Protein: 3.6g, Carbs: 39.5g, Fats: 3.6g

## 6. Warm Barley Cereal with Strawberries

**Ingredients:**

1 cup of quick-cooking barley

3 cups of skim milk

1 tbsp of ground flax meal

¼ tsp of salt

¼ cup of strawberry jam

4-5 fresh strawberries, sliced

1 tbsp of almonds, chopped

**Preparation:**

In a large saucepan, stir together quick-cooking barley, skim milk, one tablespoon of ground flax meal, and salt. Bring to a boil and reduce the heat to medium. Simmer for ten minutes. Remove from the heat and cool for a while.

Stir in strawberry jam and almonds. Top with fresh strawberries and serve.

Nutrition information per serving: Kcal: 122, Protein: 2.5g, Carbs: 26.7g, Fats: 1.8g

## 7. Creamy Baked Zucchini with Thyme

**Ingredients:**

1 medium-sized zucchini, sliced into one inch thick slices

2 large tomatoes, sliced into one inch thick slices

1 large red bell pepper, sliced into one inch thick slices

5 tbsp of Greek yogurt

1 garlic clove, crushed

1 tsp of dried thyme

3 whole eggs

3 tbsp of whole milk

1 ½ tbsp of parmesan cheese, grated

½ tsp of salt

¼ tsp of pepper

3 tbsp of olive oil

**Preparation:**

Preheat the oven to 350 degrees.

Grease one (9x13-inch) casserole pan with olive oil and set aside.

In a small bowl, stir together Greek yogurt, crushed garlic, and parmesan cheese.

In another bowl, whisk together eggs, milk, and dred thyme.

Now place zucchini in a casserole dish. Make another layer with tomatoes, and finish with red bell pepper. Spread Greek yogurt mixture over it and bake for 30 minutes.

Remove from the oven and gently spread the egg mixture using a kitchen brush.

Place in the oven for 3 more minutes and serve.

Nutrition information per serving: Kcal: 150, Protein: 7.9g, Carbs: 7.3g, Fats: 12.2g

### 8. Warm Mussel Risotto with Rosemary

**Ingredients:**

1 cup of rice

7oz mussels

1 small onion, finely chopped

1 garlic clove, crushed

1 tbsp of dry rosemary, finely chopped

¼ cup of salted capers

1 tsp of chili pepper, ground

½ tsp of salt

3 tbsp of olive oil

4 salted anchovies

**Preparation:**

Place the rice in a deep pot. Add three cups of water and bring it to a boil. Cook for 15 minutes, stirring occasionally.

Heat up the olive oil over medium heat. Add finely chopped onion and garlic. Stir-fry until translucent. Now add the mussels, rosemary, chili pepper, and salt. Continue to cook for 7-10 minutes. Remove from the heat and combine with rice.

Add capers, top with anchovies, and mix well.

Serve!

Nutrition information per serving: Kcal: 187 Protein: 4g, Carbs: 39g, Fats: 17g

### 9. Cold Tomato Couscous

**Ingredients:**

5 oz of couscous

3 tbsp of tomato sauce

3 tbsp of lemon juice

1 small-sized onion, chopped

1 cup of vegetable stock

½ small-sized cucumber,sliced

½ small-sized carrot, sliced

¼ tsp of chili powder

¼ tsp of salt

¼ tsp of black pepper

3 tbsp of olive oil

½ cup of fresh parsley, chopped

**Preparation:**

First, pour the couscous into a large bowl. Boil the vegetable broth and slightly add it the couscous while stirring constantly. Leave it for about 10 minutes until couscous absorbs the liquid. Cover with a lid and set aside. Stir from time to time to speed up the soaking process and break the lumps with a spoon.

Meanwhile, preheat the olive oil in a frying pan, and add the tomato sauce. Add chopped onion and stir until translucent. Set aside and let it cool for few minutes.

Add the oily tomato sauce to the couscous and stir well. Now add lemon juice,chopped parsley, chili powder, salt, and pepper to the mixture and give it a final stir.

Serve with sliced cucumber, carrot, and parsley.

Nutrition information per serving: Kcal: 261, Protein: 8.2g, Carbs: 38.8g, Fats: 7.4g

## 10. Lean Beef and Eggplant Stew

**Ingredients:**

7oz lean beef, chopped into bite sized pieces

1 eggplant, sliced

1 medium-sized onion, peeled and chopped

2 large, fresh tomatoes, roughly chopped

1 large potato, chopped

7.5 oz green beans

3.5 oz cabbage, shredded

1 medium-sized chili pepper

2 stalks of celery

3 tbsp of olive oil

1 tbsp of red wine vinegar

Salt to taste

1 tsp of sugar

½ tbsp of basil, dry

**Preparation:**

Chop the eggplants into bite-sized pieces and season with some salt. Allow it to stand for about 5 minutes and rinse well.

Meanwhile, heat up the olive oil over a medium heat. Add the onions and stir-fry for 2-3 minutes. Now add celery, basil, sugar, salt, vinegar, and tomatoes. Continue to cook for 2 more minutes.

Transfer to a deep pot and add other ingredients. Add about one cup of water and cook for about 20 minutes over high temperature.

Nutrition information per serving: Kcal: 198 Protein: 38g, Carbs: 27g, Fats: 19g

## 11. Creamy Yogurt Wraps with Ripe Tomatoes

**Ingredients:**

8oz chicken breast, boneless and skinless, cut into bite-sized pieces

½ medium-sized bell pepper, finely chopped

½ cup of red beans, cooked

3 large ripe tomatoes, roughly chopped

3 tbsp of extra-virgin olive oil

½ tsp of dry oregano

1 tsp of sugar

1 tsp of ground cumin

¼ cup of fresh parsley, finely chopped

½ cucumber, sliced

1 cup of thick yogurt

4 round tortillas (you can use pita breads instead)

**Preparation:**

Heat up the olive oil in a medium-sized skillet, over medium heat. Add chopped tomato and stir-fry for about five minutes, or until the liquid has evaporated. Now add oregano, cumin, and sugar. Mix well, cover, and set aside.

Meanwhile, heat up some more olive oil. Add chopped chicken and stir-fry for ten minutes, stirring constantly.

Sprinkle some water over each tortilla and warm them up in a microwave. If you're using pita breads, just warm them up.

Spread the tomato mixture over each tortilla and add sliced cucumber, chopped meat, bell pepper, and red beans. Top with yogurt and parsley. Serve!

Nutrition information per serving: Kcal: 270, Protein: 39g, Carbs: 31g, Fats: 13g

## 12. Sweet Potato Patties with Fig Jam

**Ingredients:**

1lb sweet potato, peeled

8oz all purpose flour plus 4oz more for dough

2oz wheat grits

1 egg yolk

2oz butter, melted

1 tsp of salt

Filling:

8oz unsweetened fig jam

4oz butter

1.5oz breadcrumbs

Other:

Powdered sugar

**Preparation:**

Gently peel the sweet potato and slice into one inch thick slices. Place in a deep pot and add enough water to cover. Bring it to a boil and cook until soften. This should take about five minutes because sweet potato takes less time to soften.

Remove from the heat and drain. Mash into a smooth puree. You can use a food processor for this to save yourself some time. Transfer to a bowl. Add 8oz flour, wheat grits, yolk, salt and butter. If you're using a food processor, the entire process will be much easier. If not, mash well with a fork and make a smooth dough-like mixture.

Roll the dough out until approximately 1-5 inches thick. Cut into 2-inches thick squares. Place one teaspoon of fig jam into each sqare, cover with another one, and tightly press the edges.

Place patties into a deep pot and add enough water to cover. Cook for 15 minutes over a medium heat. Remove from the heat and drain. Cool for a while.

Meanwhile, melt the butter in a large saucepan. Add breadcrumbs and briefly fry for 2-3 minutes.

Sprinkle breadcrumbs over patties and add some powdered sugar.

Serve.

Nutrition information per serving: Kcal: 182, Protein: 1.5g, Carbs: 27.5g, Fats: 8.4g

## 13. Slow-Cooked Ginger Chicken

**Ingredients:**

2 pounds chicken thighs (skin and bones should be left on)

1 tablespoon chili powder

Fresh basil

Black pepper, freshly ground

Sea salt

16 ounces coconut water

1 tablespoon grated ginger, fresh

1 tablespoon coriander seeds

8 peeled and lightly smashed garlic cloves

**Preparation:**

Put the chicken thighs along with garlic in the slow cooker. Add rest of the spices, sprinkling them evenly over the chicken thighs. Pour the coconut water on the thighs and add the fresh basil. Cover the slow cooker and set the heat to low. You need to cook the thighs for around 3 to 4 hours before they are tender enough to eat. The liquid will also give off an enticing aroma when the ginger chili chicken is ready.

Nutrition information per serving: Kcal: 301 Protein: 33.2g, Carbs: 3.2g, Fats: 15.4g

### 14. Southern Lamb Stew

**Ingredients:**

3lbs lamb cutlets

10 dried chilies

1 ½ tsp of salt

4 Japones chilies

1 ttbsp ground cumin

3 cups water

1 quartered large yellow onion

5 crushed garlic cloves

**Preparation:**

Take a sharp knife and slice each chili down the middle. Make sure you cut it into two neat halves so the seeds and the stems of the chilies can be removed easily. Take a small saucepan and toss the chilies into it. Put in all the spices along with the garlic and onion. Then, pour 3 cups of water into the saucepan. Turn the heat up to high and bring the mixture to a boil. Once boiled, let it cool for 10 minutes.

Take 2 cups of the mixture from the saucepan along with garlic, onion and chilies and put in a blender. Puree the mixture till it turns completely smooth. Take the lamb cutlets and put it in the pot. Pour the mixture in the blender over the cutlets, set the heat to medium and let it cook for 1 hour. Stir the sauce properly and shred the cutlets before serving.

Nutrition information per serving: Kcal: 135 Protein: 15.62g, Carbs: 5g, Fats: 8.31g

## 15. Wild Salmon Salad

Ingredients:

2 medium-sized cucumbers, sliced

A handful of Iceberg lettuce, torn

¼ cup of sweet corn

1 large tomato, roughly chopped

8oz smoked wild salmon, sliced

4 tbsp of freshly squeezed orange juice

Dressing:

1 ¼ cup of liquid yogurt, 2% fat

¼ cup of fat-free mayonnaise

1 tbsp of fresh mint, finely chopped

2 garlic cloves, crushed

1 tbsp of sesame seeds

**Preparation:**

Combine vegetables in a large bowl. Drizzle with orange juice and top with salmon slices. Set aside.

In another bowl, whisk together yogurt, mayonnaise, mint, crushed garlic, and sesame seeds.

Drizzle over salad and toss to combine. Serve cold.

Nutrition information per serving: Kcal: 521, Protein: 32.2g, Carbs: 63.5g, Fats: 24.3g

## 16. Fresh Italian Parsley Pasta with Seafood

**Ingredients:**

1 pack of any pasta you like

1 pound of frozen seafood mix

4 tbsp of olive oil

2 garlic cloves, crushed

1 small onion, peeled and finely chopped

½ tsp of dry oregano

¼ tsp of salt

¼ cup of white wine

**Preparation:**

Use the package instructions to prepare pasta. Rinse well and drain. Set aside.

Heat up the olive oil over a medium temperature. Add the onion and garlic and stir-fry for several minutes, or until translucent. Now add seafood mix, oregano, wine and salt. Reduce the heat to low and cook until the seafood mix have softened. You might want to check the octopus as it takes the most time to soften. Turn off the heat, add pasta and cover. Let it stand for 10 minutes before serving.

Nutritional values: Kcal: 315 Protein: 20g, Carbs: 42g, Fats: 8g

## 17. Pide Bread with Stewed Veggies

**Ingredients:**

7oz lean ground beef

½ small green pepper, finely chopped

½ small red bell pepper, finely chopped

1 large tomato, peeled and chopped

1 small onion, finely chopped

½ cup of grated gouda cheese

4 tbsp of extra virgin olive oil

1 tsp of cayenne pepper, ground

1 tsp of chili pepper, ground

½ tsp of salt

1 pide bread

**Preparation:**

Preheat the oven to 350 degrees.

Heat up two tablespoons of olive oil over medium temperature. Stir-fry the onion for 2 minutes and add finely chopped green and red pepper. Continue to cook for one more minute and add meat. Cook for ten minutes and remove from the heat.

Spread the meat mixture over the pide bread, add chopped tomato, grated gouda cheese, cayenne pepper, chili pepper, and salt. Top with two tablespoons of olive oil and bake for 5 minutes.

Serve warm.

Nutrition information per serving: Kcal: 369, Protein: 30g, Carbs: 58g, Fats: 24g

## 18. Ground Beef Cannelloni

**Ingredients:**

1 pack of cannelloni (8.8oz)

2 medium-sized red onions, finely chopped

1 pound of lean ground beef

½ tsp of salt

¼ tsp of freshly ground black pepper

3 tbsp of vegetable oil

**Preparation:**

Heat up the vegetable oil over a medium temperature. Stir-fry the onions for 3 minutes and add ground beef. Stir well and continue to cook for another ten minutes. Use the mixture to fill cannelloni.

Place in the oven for 20 minutes, or until golden brown.

Nutritional information per serving: Kcal: 417, Protein: 47g, Carbs: 43.5g, Fats: 24g

## 19. Lean Spring Stew

**Ingredients:**

1 pound diced fire roasted tomatoes

4 boneless & skinless chicken thighs

1 tablespoon dried basil

8 ounces chicken stock

Salt & pepper

4 ounces tomato paste

3 chopped celery stalks

3 chopped carrots

2 chili peppers, finely chopped

2 tablespoons olive oil

1 finely chopped onion

2 garlic cloves, crushed

½ container mushrooms

Sour cream

**Preparation:**

Heat up the olive oil over a medium-high temperature. Add the celery, onions and carrots and stir-fry for 5 to 10 minutes. Transfer to a deep pot and add tomato paste, basil, garlic, mushrooms and seasoning. Keep stirring the vegetables till they are completely covered by tomato sauce. At the same time, cut the chicken into small cubes to make it easier to eat.

Put the chicken in a deep pot, pour the chicken stock over it and throw in the tomatoes. Stir the chicken in to ensure the ingredients and vegetables are properly mixed with it. Turn the heat to low and cook for about an hour. The vegetables and chicken should be cooked through before you turn the heat off. Top with sour cream and serve!

Nutrition information per serving: Kcal: 291Protein:27g, Carbs: 37g, Fats: 3g

## 20. Stewed Beef with Olives

**Ingredients:**

2 pounds of ground beef

1 onion, peeled and chopped

2 chili peppers, finely chopped and seeds removed

3 garlic cloves, crushed

2 tsp of cumin, ground

2 tbsp of apple cider vinegar

28 oz of fire-roasted tomatoes

Salt to taste

½ tsp of cinnamon, ground

Oil for frying

For serving:

¼ cup of green olives

1 tbsp of raisins

1 tbsp of toasted almonds

**Preparation:**

Heat up about three tablespoons of oil over a medium-high temperature. Add garlic, onion and chili peppers. Stir-fry for about five minutes and add cumin and cinnamon. Mix well and cook for another minute.

Season the meat with some salt and place in a frying skillet. Stir-fry for several minutes and then add other ingredients. Bring it to a boil and reduce the heat. Simmer for about 10 minutes.

Top with green olives, toasted almonds and raisins.

Nutrition information per serving: Kcal: 521 Protein: 38g, Carbs: 29.5g, Fats: 15g

## 21. Red Orange Salad

**Ingredients:**

Fresh lettuce leaves, rinsed

1 small cucumber sliced

½ red bell pepper, sliced

1 cup of frozen seafood mix

1 onion, peeled and finely chopped

3 garlic cloves, crushed

¼ cup of fresh orange juice

5 tbsp of extra virgin olive oil

Salt to taste

**Preparation:**

Heat up 3 tbsp of extra virgin olive oil over medium-high temperature. Add chopped onion and crushed garlic. Stir fry for about 5 minutes. Reduce the heat to minimum and add 1 cup of frozen seafood mix. Cover and cook for about 15 minutes, until soft. Remove from the heat and allow it to cool for a while.

Meanwhile, combine the vegetables in a bowl. Add the remaining 2 tbsp of olive oil, fresh orange juice and little salt. Toss well to combine.

Top with seafood mix and serve immediately.

Nutrition information per serving: Kcal: 286, Protein: 34.5g, Carbs: 28g, Fats: 26g

## 22. Lean Beef Rolls

**Ingredients:**

1 cup of rice

1 pound of ground beef

¼ cup of finely chopped tomato

¼ cup of finely chopped red bell pepper

1 tbsp of tomato paste

1 tbsp of chili pepper, ground

1 chili pepper, finely diced

½ tsp of salt

¼ tsp of pepper

1 tbsp of fresh lime juice

1 bunch of collard greens

1 cup of cream for serving

1 tbsp of butter

**Preparation:**

Briefly boil the collard greens (2 minutes will be enough). Remove from the heat and drain. Set aside.

Meanwhile, in a large bowl combine the ingredients and mix well. Use one tbsp of this mixture for each roll. Melt the butter in a deep pot and place the rolls. Add about ¼ cup of water, cover the pot and cook for about 30 minutes over medium temperature.

Serve with cream, cheese or yogurt.

Nutrition information per serving: Kcal: 151 Protein: 49g, Carbs: 19.1g, Fats: 9g

### 23. Cliantro Bean Salad

**Ingredients:**

1 cup of cooked beans

½ cup of sweet corn

3 spring onions, chopped

¼ small chili pepper, finely chopped

¼ tsp of cliantro

½ tsp of red wine vinegar

1 tsp of fresh lemon juice

3 tbsp of extra-virgin olive oil

A pinch of salt

**Preparation:**

In a small bowl, combine the olive oil with red wine vinegar, fresh lemon juice, cliantro, and a pinch of salt. Mix well and use to season the other ingredients.

Serve!

Nutrition information per serving: Kcal: 151 Protein: 49g, Carbs: 19.1g, Fats: 9g

## 24. Chili Salad with Peppers

**Ingredients:**

1 cup of white beans

1 red bell pepper, chopped

1 tsp of ground chili pepper

1 tsp of parsley, finely chopped

1 tbsp of olive oil

1 tsp of lemon juice

½ tsp of sea salt

**Preparation:**

Wash and peel the pepper. Chop into bite size pieces. Mix with beans in a large bowl and top with olive oil, lemon juice and salt. Serve cold.

Nutrition information per serving: Kcal: 95 Protein: 5.9g, Carbs: 11.8g, Fats: 5g

### 25. Leafy Chicken Breast Salad

**Ingredients:**

1 piece of chicken breast, 0.5 inch thick, boneless and skinless

1 cup of finely chopped lettuce

Several spinach leaves

½ cup of beans, pre-cooked

1 tbsp of fresh lime juice

1 tsp of ground chili

1 tbsp of vegetable oil

Pinch of salt

**Preparation:**

Preheat a non-stick grill pan over a medium-high temperature. Wash and pat dry the meat using a kitchen paper. Grill for about 4-5 minutes on each side. You can use some water if necessary. Several tablespoons at a time will be enough to make the process easier. Remove from the heat and cut into several pieces.

Combine the meat with other ingredients, toss with vegetable oil, fresh lime juice, and a pinch of salt. Serve.

Nutrition information per serving: Kcal: 189 Protein: 31g, Carbs: 24g, Fats: 12g

## 26. Northern Bean Soup

**Ingredients:**

1 pound of dried great northern beans

¾ cup of onions, peeled and finely chopped

½ tbsp of vegetable oil

½ tbsp of cumin, ground

½ tbps of oregano, dry

Salt and pepper to taste

4 cups of chicken broth

1 garlic clove, crushed

1 pound of chicken breast, boneless and skinless

4 ounce can of green chillies, chopped

**Preparation:**

Place the beans in a deep pot. Add enough water to cover and bring it to a boil. Cook for several minutes and remove from the heat. Cover and let it stand for several hours until soften. Drain and rinse well.

Heat up some oil in a frying skillet. Add the onion and stir-fry for about one minute. Now add the beans, crushed garlic and chicken broth. Reduce the heat and cook for about two hours.

Preheat the oven to 350 degrees. Place the ingredients in a baking dish and coat well. Cover and cook for about an hour. Serve warm.

Nutrition information per serving: Kcal: 111 Protein: 8.1g, Carbs: 25.4g, Fats: 8g

## 27. Cliantro Lentil Stew with Carrots

**Ingredients:**

10oz lentils

1.5 tbsp of butter

1 medium-sized carrot, peeled and sliced

1 small potato, peeled and chopped

1 bay leaf

¼ cup of parsley, finely chopped

½ tbsp of fresh cliantro

Salt to taste

**Preparation:**

Melt the butter in a medium-sized skillet. Add sliced carrot, chopped potato and parsley. Mix well and stir-fry for about five minutes.

Now add the lentils, 1 bay leaf, some salt and cliantro. Add about 4 cups of water and bring it to a boil. Reduce the heat, cover and cook until the lentils soften.

Sprinkle with some parsley before serving.

Nutrition information per serving: Kcal: 313 Protein: 36g, Carbs: 42.1g, Fats: 28g

## 28. Lean Spring Veggie Risotto

**Ingredients:**

1 cup of rice

½ cup of green beans, pre-cooked

2 medium-sized red bell peppers, finely chopped

1 medium-sized zucchini, sliced

1 pice of chicken breast, boneless and skinless

3 tbsp of extra virgin olive oil

½ tsp of salt

**Preparation:**

Place the rice in a deep pot. Add 2 cups of water and bring it to a boil. Reduce the heat and cook until the water evaporates. Stir occasionally.

Stir in the olive oil, salt, sliced zucchini, green beans, and peppers. Add one cup of water and continue to cook for another 10 minutes.

Meanwhile, heat up a non-stick frying pan. Place the chicken breast and cover. Cook for 15 minutes, or until the meat has softened. Serve with rice.

Nutrition information per serving: Kcal: 220 Protein: 8g, Carbs: 45g, Fats: 3g

### 29. Sweet Pumpkin Soup

**Ingredients:**

21oz sweet pumpkin meat, chopped

2 medium-sized onions, peeled and finely chopped

1 garlic clove

1 red pepper, finely chopped

1 tbsp of fresh tomato sauce

½ tbsp of chili powder

2 bay leaves

2 cups of red wine

1 cup of water

1 tsp of thyme, dry

Salt and pepper to taste

Oil for frying

**Preparation:**

Heat up some oil in a frying skillet and add the chopped onions. Stir-fry for two minutes and add finely chopped red pepper, tomato sauce, and chili powder. Continue to fry until the peper has softened. Add the remaining ingredients and bring it to a boil. Reduce the heat to minimum and cook for about an hour.

Remove from the heat and serve.

Nutrition information per serving: Kcal: 130 Protein: 24g, Carbs: 29g, Fats: 11g

## 30. Almond Rice with Beans

**Ingredients:**

3 tbsp of olive oil

2 tbsp of vegetable oil

1 small onion, peeled and chopped

3 garlic cloves, crushed

28oz beans, pre-cooked

1 tsp of dry marjoram

1 small chili pepper, finely chopped

3 tbsp of Worcestershire sauce

1.7oz toasted almonds, chopped

A handful of pumpkin seeds for serving

1 cup of cooked rice, for serving

**Preparation:**

Combine the olive oil with vegetable oil and heat up over a medium-high temperature. Add chopped onion and garlic cloves. Stir-fry for 2-3 minutes and other ingredients. Pour about ¼ cup of water and cook for about 10 minutes, or until all the water has evaporated.

Remove from the heat and chill for a while. Serve with rice and top with pumpkin seeds.

Nutrition information per serving: Kcal: 113 Protein: 17g, Carbs: 35g, Fats: 16g

### 31. Vegetarian Pea Stew

**Ingredients:**

21oz peas, pre-cooked

1 medium-sized tomato, roughly chopped

1 medium-sized onion, peeled and sliced

2 large carrots, peeled and sliced

2 small potatoes, peeled and chopped

1 celery stalk

A handful of parsley, finely chopped

2 garlic cloves, crushed

2 bay leaves

4 tbsp of fresh tomato sauce

Olive oil

**Preparation:**

Preheat some olive oil over a medium-high temperature. Add the chopped onion and garlic. Stir-fry for several minutes and add the sliced carrot, fresh tomato paste and finely chopped celery. Cook for about ten minutes, stirring constantly. Reduce the heat to minimum and add other ingredients. Pour in about 4 cups of water and cover. Cook for about 45 minutes.

Serve warm.

Nutrition information per serving: Kcal: 186 Protein: 22g, Carbs: 38g, Fats: 23g

## 32. Spicy Roasted Chicken Legs

**Ingredients:**

1lb chicken legs

1 cup of vegetable oil

1 tsp Cayenne pepper

1 tsp salt

1 tbsp dried rosemary, crushed

1 tbsp peppercorns

1 tsp brown sugar

**Preparation:**

Combine the spices with vegetable oil. Wash and pat dry chicken legs and soak them in this mixture. Refrigerate for about an hour.

Preheat the oven to 300 degrees.

Use some of the marinade to grease the baking sheet. Place the chicken legs, skin side up and cover with foil.

Roast for about an hour and remove the foil. Return to the oven and roast for another 15 minutes.

Nutrition information per serving: Kcal: 350 Protein: 51g, Carbs: 0g, Fats: 15g

## 33. Orange Arugula Salad with Smoked Turkey

**Ingredients:**

3.5 oz arugula, torn

3.5 oz lamb's lettuce, torn

3.5 oz lettuce, torn

8 oz smoked turkey breast, chopped into bite-sized pieces

2 large oranges, peeled and sliced

For dressing:

¼ cup of Greek yogurt

3 tbsp of lemon juice

1 tsp of apple cider vinegar

¼ cup of olive oil

**Preparation:**

Combine vegetables in a large bowl. Add turkey breast and toss well. Now add sliced oranges and set aside.

Place Greek yogurt in a small bowl. Add lemon juice, apple cider, and olive oil. Whisk together until fully combined.

Drizzle over salad and serve.

Nutrition information per serving: Kcal: 271, Protein: 25.3g, Carbs: 21.8g, Fats: 7.5g

### 34. Avocado Detox Smoothie

**Ingredients:**

½ avocado, peeled and roughly chopped

1 banana, peeled and chopped

Handful of baby spinach, torn

1 tbsp of honey

1 tsp of turmeric, ground

1 tbsp of flaxseed, ground

1 tbsp of goji berries

**Preparation:**

Place the ingredients in a blender and mix well for 20 seconds.

Serve cold.

Nutrition information per serving: Kcal: 298, Protein: 4.2g, Carbs: 35.6g, Fats: 0.9g

## 35. Sweet Melon Salad with Hazelnuts

**Ingredients:**

2oz toasted hazelnuts, chopped

1lb melon, cut into bite-sized pieces

3.5 oz fresh arugula, torn

5 oz fresh raspberries

Dressing:

3.5 oz fresh raspberries

3 tbsp of fresh lime juice

1 tbsp of vanilla sugar

3 tbsp of hazelnut oil

**Preparation:**

Combine melon, arugula, raspberries, and hazelnuts in a large bowl.

Place all dressing ingredients in a food processor. Pulse to combine and drizzle over salad.

Serve cold.

Nutrition information per serving: Kcal: 87, Protein: 0.8g, Carb 15.3g, Fats: 0.4g

## 36. Marinated Turkey Breast

**Ingredients:**

1lb turkey breast, boneless and skinless

1 tbsp of olive oil

4 garlic cloves

2 tbsp of apple cider vinegar

5 tbsp of fresh parsley, finely chopped

1 tsp of oregano

½ tsp of salt

**Preparation:**

Wash and pat dry the meat. Set aside.

Combine all other ingredients in a large bowl. Place the meat in it and marinate for about an hour.

Preheat the grill pan and grill the meat for about ten minutes on each side. A good idea is to add some of the marinade while grilling – about one tablespoon will be enough.

Serve immediately.

Nutrition information per serving: Kcal: 131, Protein: 21.4g, Carb 3.7g, Fats: 3.5g

### 37. Oven Roasted Beans

**Ingredients:**

24oz beans, pre-cooked

1 large onion, peeled and finely chopped

2 spring onions, finely chopped

3 cloves of garlic, crushed

2 carrots, peeled and sliced

2 tbsp of ground chili

1 tbsp of ground turmeric

**Preparation:**

Preheat the oven to 350 degrees.

Combine the ingredients in a casserole dish. Add about three cups of water and mix well. Bake for 30 minutes.

Nutrition information per serving: Kcal: 180 Protein: 24g, Carbs: 32g, Fats: 21g

## 38. Sweet Corn Quinoa with Lime Juice

**Ingredients:**

2 tbsp of olive oil

2 cloves of garlic, crushed

1 jalapeño chili pepper, finely chopped

1 cup of quinoa

1 cup of green beans, pre-cooked

1 medium-sized tomato, finely chopped

1 cup of sweet corn

1 tsp of cayenne pepper

1 avocado, peeled and cored

1 lime, juiced

A hanful of fresh coriander

Salt and pepper to taste

**Preparation:**

Preheat the olive oil over a medium temperature. Add finely chopped jalapeño chili pepper and garlic. Stir-fry for about one minute.

Now add quinoa, green beans, finely chopped tomato, corn, and chili powder. Reduce the heat and cover. Cook for about 20 minutes.

Meanwhile, clean the avocado and chop into bite-sized pieces. Combine with lime juice and fresh coriander. Add to the mixture and serve.

Nutrition information per serving: Kcal: 374 Protein: 31g, Carbs: 64g, Fats: 28g

## 39. Citrus Spring Salad

**Ingredients:**

1 small onion, peeled and finely chopped

2 medium-sized tomatoes, chopped

1 cup of fresh cliantro, finely chopped

2 cups of tuna, drained

1 medium-sized lime, juiced

¼ tsp of sea salt

1/8 tsp of freshly ground black pepper

**Preparation:**

Combine tomatoes, cheese, onions, and cliantro in a large bowl. Stir in the lime juice and toss to combine.

Flake tuna into small pieces and season with salt and pepper. Place in a bowl.

Gently toss to evenly distribute the ingredients and serve.

Nutrition information per serving: Kcal: 165, Protein: 2.1g, Carb 17.5g, Fats: 11.2g

### 40. Easy Rye Bread

**Ingredients:**

1 cup of integral wheat flour

1 cup of rye flour

½ cup of all-purpose flour

2 tsp of dry yeast

1 ½ cup of warm water

2 tbsp of extra virgin olive oil

1 tbsp of honey

1 tsp of salt

¼ cup of flaxseed

**Preparation:**

Combine all dry ingredients in a large bowl. Gradually add warm water, stirring constantly with an electric mixer on high. Now add honey and continue to mix until you have smooth dough.

Shape the bread and cover with a kitchen cloth. Let it stand for about an hour at a room temperature.

Preheat the oven to 350 degrees.

Transfer the bread to a baking sheet and bake for 45 minutes.

Let it cool before serving.

Nutrition information per serving: Kcal: 83, Protein: 3.2g, Carb 15.4g, Fats: 1.2g

# ADDITIONAL TITLES FROM THIS AUTHOR

70 Effective Meal Recipes to Prevent and Solve Being Overweight: Burn Fat Fast by Using Proper Dieting and Smart Nutrition

By

Joe Correa CSN


48 Acne Solving Meal Recipes: The Fast and Natural Path to Fixing Your Acne Problems in Less Than 10 Days!

By

Joe Correa CSN


41 Alzheimer's Preventing Meal Recipes: Reduce or Eliminate Your Alzheimer's Condition in 30 Days or Less!

By

Joe Correa CSN


70 Effective Breast Cancer Meal Recipes: Prevent and Fight Breast Cancer with Smart Nutrition and Powerful Foods

By

Joe Correa CSN